BONITA.

CHEERS TO
MARTISPALOOZA
2023 !

XOXO
MARIA

9/26/23

Bonita,

CHEERS TO
INTERSPACE
2023 !
D

LUCKY
NANCY

First Printing, 2018
Wild Cabbage Books
wildcabbagebooks.com

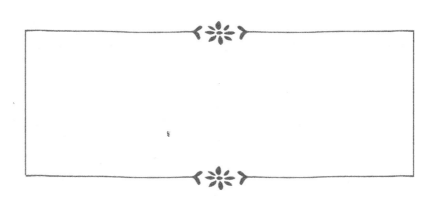

Be happy for this moment. This
moment is your life.

- Omar Kayyam

_____

_____

_____

_____

_____

_____

_____

_____

_____

_____

_____

_____

_____

_____

_____

_____

_____

_____

_____

_____

_____

_____

_____

_____

_____

-❬✳❭-

This above all: to thine ownself be true.

– Shakespeare

-❬✳❭-

Excellence is not an act, but a habit.

- Aristotle

No act of kindness, no matter how small, is ever wasted.
— Aesop

The way to be happy is to make others so.

- Robert Ingersoll

Each of us is limitless; each of us with his
or her right upon the earth.

– Walt Whitman

Peace is always beautiful.

— Walt Whitman

The greatest mistake you can make in life
is to be continually fearing you will make
one.

— Elbert Hubbard

Bloom where you are planted.

— 1 Corinthians KJV